ACCEPTANCE

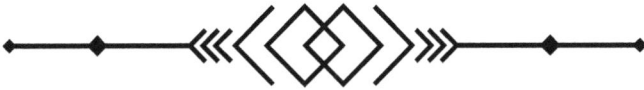

THE LANGUAGE
OF RECOVERY

Jeff Rounds

First Paperback Edition August 2024

Cover and Interior Design by The Deliberate Page

Paperback ISBN: 979-8-9911959-0-4
eBook ISBN: 979-8-9911959-1-1

Library of Congress Control Number: 2024915284

Published by Jeff Rounds
mixedrecovery@gmail.com
www.mixedrecovery.com

I dedicate this book to my friends in recovery, especially three ladies who stood by me, believed in me, and saw my value while the experts did not. From 2019 through 2022, I worked with a team of mental health professionals on a self-awareness project. We were in the process of creating and implementing an online tool that would be available to the general public. While they were too busy worrying about my eccentric behaviors and bipolar symptoms, a small group of untrained people recognized that I had discovered some very important, universally true things—that mental health professionals had ignored and belittled.

Special thanks to Kristen T., Melissa S., Julie C., Don H., and the amazing people at the PC Alano Club in Plymouth/Canton, Michigan. Also, a very special thank you to Selyna Breeze for the Rapid Transformation Therapy trauma treatments she gave me, which drastically reduced the PTSD and bipolar disorder I had been experiencing for years. Your combined efforts helped give me another chance at life.

TABLE OF CONTENTS

Preface. 1

1: What is Recovery? 3

2: The Basics of Acceptance 7

3: The Anatomy of Grieving. 9

4: Identifying the Stages of Awareness 17

5: The Toxic Cycle 23

6: Resentments and Character Defects. 31

7: The Solutions 35

8: Daily Reprieve. 45

9: Formulas and Patterns. 51

10: Pros and Cons of Recovery. 53

11: Into Action / Tips for Sponsors. .59

12: Manifesting 69

About the Author 71

PREFACE

This guide has been inspired by Alcoholics Anonymous, including the twelve steps of recovery and the article known as Acceptance.

> *"And acceptance is the answer to all my problems today. When I am disturbed, it is because I find some person, place, thing, or situation - some fact of my life - unacceptable to me. I can find no serenity until I accept that person, place, thing, or situation as being exactly the way it is supposed to be at this moment. Nothing, absolutely nothing, happens in God's world by mistake. Until I could accept my alcoholism, I could not stay sober; unless I accept life completely on life's terms, I cannot be happy. I need to concentrate not so much on what needs to be changed in the world as on what needs to be changed in me and my attitudes."*

- Alcoholics Anonymous Big Book, Fourth Edition, p417

This book's premise is that acceptance truly is the answer to all personal issues and that having a deeper understanding of acceptance leads to higher levels of inner peace, personal balance, and a sense of purpose. When we undertake to learn, practice, give, and receive acceptance, we create a safe atmosphere for healing and speaking freely. The primary goal of this guide is to increase self-awareness and impact humanity in a positive manner, encouraging complete balance, wellness, and acceptance for all.

I recommend purchasing or acquiring the *Alcoholics Anonymous Big Book*, which is referenced a number of times in this guide.

Please note: many of the expressions in this book are not supported by science or formal education and may be in conflict with clinical definitions. As one example and for the sake of humanity, the Freudian model of Ego has been rejected completely. Also, this guide offers a more recovery-based understanding of the grieving process as compared to the well-known and incomplete Kubler-Ross model. I used methods some might consider unorthodox to gather the data presented in this guide, and though I offered these findings to a professional community, they were ignored. Three years of my efforts were wasted in an attempt to teach recovery to psychology professionals.

Though each has its place (professional and amateur), this guide is based entirely on the items that are public domain and considered to be universal truths, meaning they apply to all humans. My writing style is minimalist and is intended to remove as much presence of Ego as possible, leaving only honest and relatable statements.

If you are in need of support and/or are interested in becoming peer support for others, please contact mixedrecovery@gmail.com or visit our website, www.mixedrecovery.com, for more information. Mixed Recovery, Inc. is a for-profit company that provides both paid support to the general public and unpaid support for people actively involved in twelve step recovery programs.

1
WHAT IS RECOVERY?

There are thousands of peer support groups, both with and without twelve-step style recovery, worldwide. There are also numerous programs that train recovery for a variety of conditions. With a growing industry and an obvious need for people to express themselves in healthy, safe environments, recovery programs are some of the safest ways to accommodate this need.

Anyone capable of listening without judging, steering, or enabling another person qualifies to give healthy peer support. People with experience in completing a recovery program are also best suited to sponsor other people through the process of recovery. Steering is using our personal values to guide or control others; enabling is doing for others what they can and need to be doing for themselves. Healthy sponsorship includes boundaries that prevent these behaviors and practicing detachment keeps us from harming ourselves in the process of supporting others.

People need to express themselves in a variety of ways. The healthiest people are generally those who are comfortable expressing themselves honestly in all situations. This behavior illustrates high levels of acceptance, self-awareness, and the presence of adaptive coping skills.

Adversely, many people learn to hide their feelings and that there are penalties for expressing themselves. In time, this repression of feelings increases causing more damage to our mental health. Much of human behavior is shame-based and results from a process called Social Conditioning. This process often traumatizes people into behaving unnaturally, resulting in more fear-based thinking and greater levels of stress. Social Conditioning is essentially using shame to control and assimilate others into their surroundings. Shame causes trauma while creating lasting and recognizable patterns in human behavior. Recovery means recovering the unconditioned self, first by identifying harmful behaviors and patterns caused by shame, then applying a process of healing and making amends (replacing harmful behaviors). It is possible to increase self-awareness, emotional intelligence, and acceptance through recovery. Traumas do not need to be catastrophic or unbearable experiences. Trauma is simply defined as any amount of shame that is trapped in our systems. The complete variety of human traumas can be easily described as falling under two categories: resentments and character defects.

Resentment is a "re-sent-ment," meaning each time we think about something, it has a negative impact on us, resulting in either anger or depression. Character defects are the reasons why we hold onto resentments; they are the things we judge about ourselves or others as bad, evil or wrong. Through open communication and the recovery process, these traumas can be inventoried, discussed, released, and healed, thus becoming strengths and virtues that are useful in helping others.

This Mixed Recovery, Inc. program was created to share some of the more effective aspects of recovery. Also, information will be provided to help identify the pitfalls of recovery and how to avoid becoming an enabler trapped in a toxic cycle with a sponsee or client. Knowing how to create and maintain healthy boundaries prevents sponsorship from becoming draining. Being safe for someone else requires becoming vulnerable and risking emotional pain; with awareness and training, recovery sponsorship can remain positive for all parties.

2
THE BASICS OF ACCEPTANCE

Humans have many needs; one often neglected is the nurturing we receive when we experience acceptance. One principle of this training program is that people with similar life experiences are often best suited to give others emotional support and acceptance. Emotional support does not require clinical training or lengthy courses and is often best accomplished with less structure. One major benefit of remaining nonprofessional is that sponsors are generally available to give support at any or most times without an appointment. Life is unpredictable, and sponsors are often more accessible and able to give support during crises than mental health professionals.

Caring for others in a healthy manner requires that we are aware of our shortcomings and actively check ourselves for honesty and integrity. Many people who are drawn to helping others may have codependency issues and are susceptible to toxic relationships. Practicing detachment, maintaining boundaries, and being mindful of approval-seeking can help protect sponsors from over-investing. Being honest, self-aware, empathetic, and accountable are positive qualities to aid those who are suffering. The acceptance people receive in recovery can be life-changing. Also, knowing the stages of grieving intimately is very useful in guiding people to reach acceptance. Awareness of the stages of grieving can provide the information needed to communicate safely without causing others to become defensive and lose faith in the process.

The most useful tool for anyone in a support role is the ability to listen completely to others without any desire to judge what is being said. The goal of an effective listener is to relate to and mirror the other person in a sincere, healthy manner. Listening is near impossible when our minds are filled with thoughts of our own or desire to make a point. Sometimes, being useful means making no points, possibly saying very few things, if any. Giving acceptance is, in many ways, an act of love. Love, in its purest form, is 100 percent acceptance and contains no emotional signature at all. Being able to accept someone no matter what they are saying, thinking, feeling, and doing is a virtue that requires practice. In recovery, trust is broken, and the process generally ends when people sense they are being judged and not accepted.

To help people create a safe atmosphere for other people, this training program presents concepts of universal truth found in Buddhism, twelve-step recovery, philosophy, and world religion. The terms are NOT clinical; they are intended to be simple, clear, and comprehensive. The term attachment is used excessively and refers to all emotional experiences. Ego (logic, will, and desire) is the collection of all attachments; for many, it represents their concept of self. The authentic self exists outside the world of thoughts and feelings and is always peaceful, the witness of our lives. We, the witnesses, are not our thoughts, we are not the mind, we are not the body, and we are not any of the labels that have been placed on us. At a core level, the real self is peace, and everything that is not peaceful is Ego and, ultimately, the cause of all suffering.

3
THE ANATOMY OF GRIEVING

For the sake of clarity, it is important to understand certain universal truths in terms of Buddha's teachings. The Buddha spoke in the truth of self-awareness and explained that "Attachment is the root of all Suffering." He went on to explain that "Life is Suffering," which is to say that, at least for humans, life is not possible without attachments and having emotional attachments to material world experiences causes suffering. Attachment is ALL experiences that hold an emotional signature. Note that in every moment of our lives, whatever we are experiencing is being recorded in our subconscious mind. These experiences are interconnected with our emotions, thoughts, and behaviors. Wherever we are emotionally invested, we are attached, and the more we are invested, the more we will suffer when the attachment is lost, broken, or challenged. Being attached creates the first stage of grieving: denial. Without our awareness, every human is in denial of something because we are all attached to something, a very simple and closed system. Having an emotional signature of zero or nothing represents the peace that comes with having no thoughts or emotions invested. People can be peaceful when in denial; if an attachment is lost, they are not peaceful again until they reach acceptance. Both Denial in its unchallenged state and Acceptance can be peaceful; only when an attachment is lost, broken, or challenged do we become aware of whether this peace is the result of denial or acceptance.

Acceptance can be faked or falsely induced using repression, willful ignorance, different forms of manipulation, or therapeutic conditioning. Superficial therapies such as EMDR (Eye Movement Desensitization and Reprocessing) and NLP (Neuro-Linguistic Programming) may reprogram an attachment as less harmful. However, this is often a repression, not an expression of suffering. Induced peace lacks the emotional intelligence and complete understanding that can only result from surrendering to our emotions and processing a loss. Breaking an attachment means changing our minds through completing the grieving process.

At the core of every attachment is the emotional signature of shame. The peaceful, "spiritual" part of us knows better than to become attached because we recognize the harm it causes. That knowing part of us is the conscience that guides and heals us. The more we ignore it, the more shame the attachment accumulates and the more harm it causes. Life is finite and we all desire a life of comfort and pleasures without consequences. We tend to reject the reality that life is not kind, fair, or just and nothing is promised to anyone. Without acceptance, we are blind to the complete truth that life is more peaceful without attachments. In the bargaining stage of grieving, our Ego is in conflict with the peaceful part of us and causes us to feel shame, embarrassment, anxiety, stress, depression, and anger. In surrender, we judge and punish ourselves, asking ourselves "why" as we let go of the logic, will, and desire to have something we want. Completing the grieving process is a loss of self and the awareness that although we cannot have what we want, life will be manageable anyway. Acceptance cannot be reached without surrender, often leading to crying, which many people fear and avoid. People have often been conditioned to hide, repress, and bury their tears, which only increases the amount of shame, aka trauma we carry. In reality, crying is the most effective way to release trauma and the most direct path to gaining more acceptance.

This book presents a model of grieving that varies from the Kubler-Ross model and is based more on personal experience combined with knowledge of twelve-step recovery.

KUBLER-ROSS STAGES OF GRIEVING

1. Denial
2. Anger
3. Bargaining
4. Depression
5. Acceptance

ACTUAL GRIEVING

1. **Denial** – Unknowingly or willfully unaware of the presence of harm.
2. **Bargaining** – Logic used to defend an attachment, thoughts that generate anger, anxiety, depression, and a continued state of non-acceptance.
3. **Surrender** – Letting go of control, allowing ourselves to feel every emotion no matter how painful.
4. **Acceptance** – Peace. The highest form of intelligence and understanding, free from emotional attachment.

Denial – Denial is a sincere state of mind. In denial, people do not see the harm in their attachments, which shows in their thoughts, beliefs, words, and behaviors. To a mind in denial, the way we live makes sense, and there is no need for change. We also tend to believe that we are right and that when negative things occur in our lives, it is not our fault, and we assign blame to something or someone else.

Also, in denial, people tend to brag and exhibit the traits common to narcissism. The more denial a person accumulates, the more they self-identify with their Ego (logic, will, and desire) and lose a connection to life's spiritual, intuitive, honest, and self-aware dimensions.

Every human is in denial about something. In fact, people who are offended by that statement are proof of the statement; all defensive responses, all anger and depression indicate denial that has been triggered and the bargaining stage of grieving. Anything that triggers us shows where we are attached. However, we need attachments to function as humans because without logic, will, and desire, a human would simply lay still and die, action would be pointless, and life would have no meaning. Life with zero attachments is likely impossible for humans and many living things. Using Buddhist monks as examples of having few attachments, the act of living a peaceful, simple life and denying worldly desires still requires a collection of attachments.

Denial can become a natural reflex to many things. Like exercising a muscle, people practice lying to each other and themselves, unable to face or express their honest feelings out of fear. We have the option of creating willful denial in ourselves, making excuses that minimize the known presence of harm with a paradoxical equation: "It is not that bad." When examined more closely at the wording, Ego reveals its true nature.

It = the Harm

is not = Denial

that bad = the measure of how bad the harm is

This statement, written in full form, reads as **"The harm is not as bad as the harm is,"** convincing us we can manage even more if needed. Without a willingness to recognize the harm, people create the most convincing arguments in their bargaining process, and the story they use to convince themselves is the one they express to others when the attachment is questioned. Example: "I know I shouldn't smoke, but it helps relax me."

Bargaining – Once denial has been exposed, humans engage their problem-solving abilities to maintain their attachments. In bargaining, people experience anger and depression in varying degrees. We tend to complain and point out flaws, expressing what we cannot accept. A challenged attachment often causes the human mind to become an excuse factory, rejecting new information. When angry, we bargain to keep what we want, and as we begin to accept the loss, we shift more into depression. Anger and depression may swing like a pendulum as our thoughts fight themselves and we process the logic of bargaining, which may last for moments, years, or even a lifetime.

It's important to note that when people express themselves with anger, they are often at their most exposed and honest, stating what they cannot accept, their most negative beliefs, excuses, threats and accusations. People also use anger to harm or manipulate others as a form of emotional abuse, exaggerating harmful values while placing shame and blame outside of themselves.

Expressing anger is needed to move through bargaining. Also, when anger is expressed, other people will sometimes accommodate our needs. However, complaining can become habitual, illustrating a mind constantly judging and experiencing thoughts of non-acceptance. People who complain and judge habitually often need the most acceptance and are least able to experience it.

It is possible to become emotionally attached to anything, including complaining. Friedrich Nietzsche speaks of how those who loathe still esteem themselves as ones who loathe.

People complain until their anger is exhausted, and they become tired of thinking about a particular issue. An issue may fall into submission unresolved and out of mind but may be exposed with questions or memories that trigger the attachment. Once we have bargained, hurt enough, and recognized that we are powerless over a loss, we become ready to enter the third stage of grieving: surrender.

Surrender – Surrender can be done willfully, or we may be forced by circumstance. In surrender, our emotions catch up to us, which is overwhelming. All the beliefs and emotions we hold now feel like punishment as we experience the shame, regret, guilt, and other fear-based consequences of loss. In surrender, we are learning and experiencing a biochemical transformation that many people would describe as a spiritual awakening. Oddly, even people with little or no faith will often say the words, "Oh God, please no... please, not again, take this from me, I cannot handle it anymore, Oh God, why?" etc.

In surrender, people become childlike and may cry, pray, and beg for death. In these moments, we may remember other times we have suffered and feel we are being measured as worthless. All of this pain reduces humans to tears, provided there is a willingness to release the tears. Some losses may require tears to be expressed numerous times, and the memories may always result in tears, although the need for grieving may diminish each time.

People rarely communicate surrender to each other; when they do, it may be tears mixed with anger, complaining and/or confessing. Once we have cried until there is nothing left to cry about and complain until all anger is exhausted, we let go of our logic, will, and desire to think about the loss and enter into the final stage of grieving and awareness known as acceptance. Each completed grieving process increases emotional intelligence, intuition, and humility. As the Ego dies, the peace-seeking part of our existence grows in understanding, leading us toward acceptance.

With great losses come great releases of energy, and crying is exhausting. Sleeping is recommended to regain balance and take a break from the bargaining mind. Because emotional pain is one of the most difficult things for humans to endure, it's important to remember that it will eventually end, and we completely lose the desire to fight. Surrender is the extreme expression of powerlessness, and it is when we are most honest with ourselves. Daily surrender may be used as a form of emotional maintenance, freeing us from the desire to overthink.

Acceptance – Acceptance is the highest level of human understanding; without it, all knowledge is just attachments. Reaching acceptance, we have emotional intelligence and have resolved any logic, will, or desire we had attached to the loss. With each lesson in acceptance, we remove the need to think about our attachments. There is no longer any desire to bargain or complain, and our explanation of the loss is short and accountable. In acceptance, there is no longer a need to express anger or depression and no desire to return to the memories that trigger negative emotions. Acceptance is experienced in degrees and can either be increased or decreased depending on how we choose to think about what we are experiencing. In general, the less we think about memories, the more peace and acceptance we can experience.

The purest forms of acceptance have no emotional signature at all and are peaceful. In acceptance, people behave selflessly while maintaining healthy boundaries. They are also more compassionate and able to avoid threats they intuitively identify. People with high levels of acceptance are proficient listeners because their minds are no longer filled with bargaining, and when they communicate, it is mostly in terms of gratitude and confession. People in acceptance are nonjudgmental and natural healers, examples of the peace they feel.

As levels of acceptance increase, so does intuition, honesty, and gratitude. A person with a mind filled with bargaining will not experience much of the world of intuition. A mind free from bargaining can learn to witness many things and avoid the pitfalls created by fear-based thinking. People in acceptance also tend to have more faith in life and less struggle. They may experience less selfish ambition, more creativity, and a constant willingness to learn. People in acceptance are easier to interact with and will not have a desire to manipulate, control, or behave selfishly. Effectively grieving losses causes people to recognize their conscience and virtues, reducing desires to cause or experience harm.

At our cores, we all have the same conscience and values, though we are often unaware because bargaining and denial block the information we all experience internally. In acceptance, everyone has the same moral code and knows the same things but has a different language to express it based on their personal life experiences.

4

IDENTIFYING THE STAGES OF AWARENESS

Whether in groups or one-on-one, it's important to recognize when people are ready, willing, and able to change. Willingness to change is directly connected to our self-awareness and where we are in the grieving process. People can be encouraged in any stage of grieving, yet it requires understanding to maintain healthy boundaries and avoid the hazards of working with people in Denial. People often need to be heard and validated and assured they have options. The challenge is to be supportive without triggering defenses.

People respond defensively to a number of perceived threats, including embarrassment, personal loss, disrespect, challenged beliefs, gaslighting, physical harm, and accusations. If a person feels judged, they will often reduce or end their willingness to be open, honest, and vulnerable.

To avoid causing a threat, learn the signs of denial and how to side with it to regain peace. Witnessing and recalling our own grieving and acceptance is a powerful tool in aiding others still experiencing suffering. Using the correct language is also important; avoid telling people what to do at all costs, replace that with explaining what has worked for you and understand that everyone's recovery looks different, even when we do the same things.

Denial has predictable symptoms, and when triggered, human defenses sound like "I do not have a problem; you do." People will often pose their most convincing arguments when denial is triggered because it engages the bargaining mind, and we tell others the same justifications and reasoning we have been telling ourselves. Become aware that every accusation is a confession. Also, the stronger the argument, the more emotionally invested the person is. When in denial, people will often project, shame, and blame towards anyone they believe to be in opposition. Denial, in many cases, is denying the emotional impact our thoughts, words, and behaviors have on ourselves and others. Denial, in the simplest terms, is a lack of emotional intelligence.

Intuitively, we know when other people are closed-minded or defensive. To minimize the damage and even reverse the process of triggering defensives, take the side of the threatened person, focusing on the healthy aspects of what is being expressed. Agree with objections and offer compassion and respect for boundaries whenever a trigger is recognized. Be willing to let someone shut down and isolate themselves while they process their feelings because the experience is often embarrassing. Some people may even tap into some dark and hateful feelings when triggered, and it could be best for everyone if they are allowed and even encouraged to express their thoughts and feelings of anger. Examples:

"I am glad you are letting this out; it's really good to express yourself."

"You are right; that sounds like it would make me angry, too."

"I can understand why you feel that way; I can relate."

"That must be difficult, and I am sorry for what you are experiencing."

These are examples of things that come naturally for people with an accumulation of acceptance. Memorizing exact wording and precise techniques will often misguide us from the intuitive responses that will come effortlessly as a result of being fully present. Study this guide as a basis for helping others and not necessarily the only or perfect way. Have faith that the right words will come if your intentions are selfless.

Denial continues during the bargaining stage, and it often sounds like complaining. Complaining is a needed part of the grieving process. Complaining to people who will listen without judging and complaining to a higher power are healthy outlets for this need. In many cases, complaining inspires needed change. Ego has a need for a sense of being right and having others sympathize with our suffering provides the acceptance and validation needed to process loss. Complaining can be very effective but it can also be very manipulative and destructive. Chronic complainers may seek people willing to rescue them, which can become very draining for anyone attempting to support them. Without boundaries and awareness, it can be very easy to enter a toxic cycle with a client, sponsee, or another person in general. It is unhealthy to give assistance if expecting change from others, especially when they are currently incapable due to denial.

People change for two main reasons and frequently a combination of both; either they have hurt enough to have let something go, or there is a promise of something bigger and better. Depending on the nature, degree, and stage of grief, change may not be possible at times and allowing someone to complain without interruption may be the best course of action. This is similar to the coddling often provided by trained professionals, and for the same reason, people in denial are unable to accept new information. A mind trapped in denial is a closed system; when triggered, it tends to shut down, and that serves no one. Eventually, if someone we are helping continues complaining, rejecting suggestions, and insisting that nothing is helping, they must be let go and considered a loss. The bottom line is that someone who refuses to change or be accountable cannot accept help because their minds are closed.

Extensive support with no hope of change is enabling and unhealthy. Also, mismatches and timing issues are common in recovery and letting go allows everyone to attract better matches. Being ineffective is emotionally draining for anyone. Whether a sponsor, mentor, coach, peer specialist or other, there is no point in forcing anything. It is not our responsibility as sponsors to fix, sell, or convince anyone of the value of taking recovery seriously; we can only help those who want it.

With a willingness to let go, we eventually grow tired of our own complaining, which naturally diminishes. When a person is closest to letting go or very near acceptance, the story and explanation of their issues become short, and they confess their feelings about the loss. When humans communicate honestly in this manner, it is an act of confession and transparency. The proper response to a confession is another honest confession. Offering advice when no question has been asked or permission given is unhealthy and considering steering. When people steer each other or give unsolicited advice, they are exhibiting their control issues and nonacceptance. The advice can be offered in the language of a confession, with the preface, "This is what has worked for me." Without qualifying a suggestion as just one possible solution, people unwittingly cross each other's boundaries, eventually creating alienation. The intention of emotional support and sponsorship is to validate the idea that everyone has their own answers, and through the confession of others, you may find yourself, hear your own story, and find your own answers.

Boundaries are an important aspect of recovery and life; they represent limits we place on ourselves. One example of a healthy boundary is accepting and reminding ourselves that every time we speak to someone about recovery, it may be the last. Practicing detachment is key in recovery because we never know the limits of another person's willingness. Honesty and self-awareness provide the intuitive information needed to maintain healthy boundaries. Body language, facial expressions, tone of voice, patterns of behavior and speech are all indicators of how receptive another person is to our support. Ego defenses protect us from perceived threats; in some cases, the imagined threats are healthy changes in our lives that we do not feel emotionally prepared to handle. Subconsciously, the mind of Ego fears letting go because it knows all losses are painful and may end in tears.

Healthy emotional support allows us to witness and encourage tears and the act of surrender as a means to gain more acceptance. How we manage another person's tears will determine how helpful and healing our support can be for them. Support means encouraging healthy behaviors and validating negative experiences while maintaining healthy boundaries. It also means listening more than we talk and avoiding the desire to give advice on personal matters. We do not tell people what they need to do; we ask them what they are willing to do and offer suggestions that have worked for us and others.

5

THE TOXIC CYCLE

Patterns and Signs – Most human behavior forms predictable patterns which can be identified with self-awareness. The subconscious mind is very powerful, and without a thought, we repeat thousands of behaviors daily, completely unaware that we have the option to change. When people become attached, that creates a state of denial, which is resistant to change. The Ego seeks comfort, stability, and effortlessness; however, life in a civilized world is none of those things. The toxic cycle can occur any time we want something we cannot have. Attached to how we want things to be, we ignore the warning signs that we are engaging in something harmful. Like a moth drawn to a hot light, the toxic cycle is one of the most common patterns of abuse, reaching every aspect of life and only requiring one person to participate, yet this pattern is especially common in romantic and financial relationships.

HOW THE TOXIC CYCLE LOOKS IN A RELATIONSHIP:

1. **Honeymoon Phase** – The toxic cycle begins with an invitation, "Welcome to my world." False positives are given,

feeding the Ego and creating the illusion of acceptance and value. "I like you, and I am like you." Often, in this stage, the victims receive some type of benefit that accommodates their deeper unresolved issues.

2. **Tensions Build** – Trouble begins as the cycle becomes less rewarding and compromises are made to accommodate the abuser. The neglected subject(s) convince themselves that "it's not that bad," and they may stay in the relationship hoping for improvement.

3. **Abuse** – An incident occurs, which may include some or all of the following:

   » Verbal Abuse
   » Accusations
   » Threats
   » Punishment
   » Disapproval
   » Gaslighting
   » Physical Harm
   » Anger and Hostility
   » Passive Aggression
   » The Silent Treatment

4. **Reconciliation** – Apologies are made with no or short-term changed behaviors. There may be empty promises made, little or no accountability mixed with excuses, gentle gaslighting, minimizing, and false positives. If effective, the process begins again, and there is another honeymoon phase.

It is important to recognize the presence of intentions and how they affect the toxic cycle. With the very best of intentions, people in denial can become very toxic to others. There are also those who genuinely intend harm because their narcissism has become sociopathic. It does not matter whether someone intends harm; the longer we remain in this cycle, the more damage it causes.

If and when things become hostile and angry words are shared, note this is when people are frequently at their most honest and reveal many things about themselves. When under verbal attack, remember that every accusation is a confession. We paint other people with our own issues and the negative outward talk is a direct reflection of the negative self-talk we are experiencing. Understand that we shame others for the qualities we cannot accept in ourselves.

> **Example:** "You are lazy and worthless" = "I struggle with a desire to be lazy, and I feel worthless, even though I tell myself I am better than you."

The toxic cycle functions very much like an addiction; the longer we stay, the more painful, difficult, and frightening it is to leave. Filled with fear, we can become attached to the idea that we cannot live without someone or something and that we are trapped because of everything we stand to lose. We regain our personal power and self-respect when we can accept all the losses and leave the situation in spite of our fears. As with everything, acceptance only occurs following surrender, and we need to let go and surrender to the feelings of loss and grief. Applying intentional grieving can give us the strength, understanding, and acceptance we need to move toward our truer selves.

The terms below describe patterns that are intertwined as parts of the toxic cycle. Identifying these patterns in ourselves and others is useful to our recovery, and learning to identify and avoid abuse can lead to more inner peace and self-respect.

The Confidence Game – Many people unwilling to change apply a technique that allows them to benefit disproportionately from the kindness of others. The toxic cycle begins with an invitation:

the promise of some reward. People who use others often start a relationship with compliments, offers, and favors, creating a false sense of security. This is called the confidence game, meaning, "I give you my confidence, and I believe in you so that later, I can abuse you." Later, when the trust is broken, the victim is blamed. With the best of intentions, people use each other with this pattern frequently.

Love Bombing – This is a variation of the confidence game, though considered more affectionate. Again, using compliments to "butter someone up" people looking for attention will create the illusion of acceptance and admiration. Sadly, these positive messages are being exaggerated for personal gain; later, negative comments will be used to maintain control or end the relationship when it no longer has any value to the abuser.

Yeah, But – When someone speaks of their problem as though they want help, then rejects all reasonable suggestions using excuses for avoiding growth, they are in an Ego trap, and it is unlikely there is anything anyone can do to help them at that moment. When we are in denial, people become excuse factories, and we tell other people all the reasons we cannot change. It is natural to say "yeah, but" when we are not ready to change.

The Roller Coaster – Addicted to drama, some people often experience mood swings, and in the absence of any real problems, they may invent some. When people have difficulty making decisions, it often means they do not yet have enough emotional information to complete the grieving process. The behaviors of people with high levels of bargaining are often erratic and confusing to others. The bargaining sounds like "maybe this or maybe that" and is represented by an inability to make and stick to decisions, which results in a rollercoaster of drama.

The Repeat Offender – Many people unable to change become chronic complainers and find that the acceptance they receive from others when they complain is enough emotional relief so they can maintain the harmful behavior indefinitely. Complaining about the same person, place, thing, or situation repeatedly is another Ego trap. This is a variation on an excuse factory.

Plausible Deniability – One of the most common forms of deceit is what some would call "white lies." Plausible deniability is creating an excuse that is convincing and reasonable, though it is not the truth at all. Some people lie constantly and seem to master the art of getting away with it simply because they present convincing lies. Recognizing the lies requires noticing how the words and behaviors do not match up. Plausible deniability is supplying a reasonable excuse for behavior that denies or minimizes harm and makes it sound like the intentions are good and not bad. Example: "I wasn't picking my nose, just scratching it."

Trapped – This is a common mentality of people in one or many toxic cycles. When the loss seems too great, people will often convince themselves that the things they are attached to are more important than they really are and those things cannot be left behind. The bargaining can be maddening for someone trying to decide how to behave when, deep down, they already know life is unmanageable for them. "I cannot leave because I will lose too much." Trapped is an illusion that can only be seen from the other side of grieving, in acceptance. The costs of staying are usually greater than any perceived loss, but until we leave the situation, it is difficult to see the truth.

The Excuse Factory – When people are unwilling to change, they have an excuse to protect every problem in their lives. They become the victim: they are not doing anything wrong; everything they try doesn't work; it is always someone else's fault. Whenever they are given a suggestion, they tell the same excuses that they have been telling themselves and expose the nonacceptance of the bargaining mind. When we are resistant to change, we will make excuses until the harm is so great, our choices are limited, and we are forced to change or remain in survival mode until we do.

Butthurt Baby – When humans are filled with shame, we can become gaslighting experts, intuitively knowing which emotions to play on so we can constantly have our needs met. When caught or challenged, people in denial will often "take their ball and go home," with an "If I can't have it, no one can" attitude. Punishing others and projecting outward is a temporary relief from shame and responsibility and empowers us as abusers until our emotions and consequences catch up to us.

Crocodile Tears – Many people can fake tears and often do so at funeral proceedings or in court. Fake tears are intended to draw concern and sympathy from other people and to present as an empathetic person when, in truth, they are overcompensating and acting. It is a common form of manipulation and an invitation to the toxic cycle.

Bully on the Playground – On rare occasions, it is possible to end a toxic cycle quickly and create an opportunity for change by setting a boundary. When someone in denial causes harm, if it is addressed immediately and with great force, they may be shamed enough to recoil and adapt. By setting boundaries and expressing dominance, we may be able to convert a bully into a friend. "I know what you are doing, and it stops now, or the relationship ends" is the ultimate message. Being ready, willing, and able to leave the relationship is a matter of self-respect. Another possibility is to approach the same situation with kindness and acceptance, setting the exact same boundary. The difference is in what feels honest to us. If we are unhealed, it is likely we need to express anger to assert ourselves. However, if we no longer possess any attachment to the behavior and have reached acceptance, the statement may sound more like this: "I know what you are doing, and I understand; I have done that myself and I do not fault you. I need to take care of myself, though, so please understand I am no longer willing to participate in that behavior."

Gold Diggers – Some people perpetually and constantly use other people. The gold digger normally has something to offer with an often-increasing price tag. Whatever they possess that is desired becomes a weapon and tool for manipulation. Sex, money, help, and support are all tools a gold digger may use to manipulate a victim and avoid personal consequences.

Damsel in Distress – This may represent the beginning of a long-term gold digger relationship, and it is not gender related. Using "crocodile tears," dramatic physical gestures, and signs of trouble to lure enablers to their rescue, the damsel in distress is another form of toxic cycle. A person who helps is now the mark in a confidence game that sounds like, "I am desperate and need help. You are so wonderful. Thank you for saving me."

Grifters – This is a term used to describe professional or habitual con artists, masters of the confidence game. Many of these people are sociopathic and lean toward criminal thinking and behavior, always looking for opportunities to apply their talents and apply the confidence game.

Smart Mouth – Some people specialize in a form of abuse that is passive-aggressive and demeaning. With a voice inflection that may sound caring and sincere, they seem to intuitively know how to say the most offensive things in disguise. Using the common tactics of gaslighting and manipulation, people who have low self-esteem focus on the faults of others and point them out, giving themselves a sense of superiority.

The High Road – Ego loves to feel self-righteous and be better than other people in some way. Having discovered a fatal flaw in another person, some people will often point out shortcoming in an attempt to bolster their own Ego. "At least I am not that bad" is the overall message, and it can be a very destructive behavior.

In order to overcome the tendency to engage in the toxic cycle, we need to identify and heal our own character defects and resentments. Only through increased awareness and willingness to change can we escape our preprogrammed patterns of harmful behavior. In most cases, it means identifying what we wanted from the toxic relationship and learning to replace that desire with one that is healthier for us.

Change often means a death of Ego, the loss of a former version of ourselves and a willingness to do something different than we have in the past. Have faith, knowing that these painful losses will end in peaceful rewards, whereas staying in a toxic cycle only guarantees more abuse and eventual abandonment.

6

RESENTMENTS AND CHARACTER DEFECTS

Resentments and character defects are closely related; they both are connected to human judgment. There are two forms of human judgment: one is Comparative Analytics, which assumes no moral position, and the other is Moral Imposition, which implies that some people can be better or know better than other people. A nonjudgmental mind acknowledges the reality that all people are equal, even though our lives are far from equal.

Moral Imposition is an unhealthy behavior, and it is present in many places, including justice systems and religions. Defining and judging the things we experience in life is an addiction for many people. With a mind filled with judgments, we are also bargaining with reality and cannot experience the peace of acceptance.

As mentioned previously, a "re-sent-ment" is any thought or memory that continues to disturb our peace each time we recall it. Also, expectation is a resentment waiting to happen, and it has a recognizable pattern. It begins with judgment and the opinion of "should." Should, shouldn't, never, always, and other absolutes rarely apply to human behavior and are generally harmful. How we think, feel, and want things to be does not matter, the most peaceful perspective is accepting the circumstances of life how they really are.

It is common for people to feel they need to do something when an experience offends their senses. In truth, we do; we need to face our worst fears and accept that we cannot always have what we want or how we want it.

In brief, resentments are any anger or depression that we hold, and our character defects are the reasons and excuses behind why we do not let them go.

Understanding resentment is best done in reverse, recalling the warning signs which led to disappointment. When we reach acceptance, it is possible to see that there were clear signs of warning, the ways we were unprotected and exposed. Ultimately, we wanted something that we could not have, ignored the warning signs, and told ourselves, "It's not that bad." The anger we feel is toward ourselves for knowing better and making harmful decisions anyway. Once an attachment is broken and we look back with acceptance, the change we need to make now becomes obvious, and we have the emotional data to reinforce this healthy decision.

> **Example:** We may know that we cannot trust someone and that we cannot afford a loss, yet we loan them money anyway. When they refuse to pay us back, the anger we feel is really not toward them; we are angry at ourselves for knowing better and trusting them anyway.

Ego has a need to be right; without a sense of right, it feels out of control and insane. To help overcome the need to be right, understand that being right is a matter of personal opinion and not universal truth. Think of any time you have been wrong in the past. Up until you realized it, you thought yourself to be right. Now, think about anything you are right about today; doesn't the same possibility exist? In reality, we are never right or wrong; we are either attached or gathering information. Making a decision about anything closes our minds to new information, leaving us vulnerable to suffering. Accepting people, places, things, and situations exactly as they are helps us to maintain a constant state of "I do not know; I wonder what this is." Without a decision, poorly invested emotions will not be spent on a lost cause.

One of the more common resentments is the one people have toward God or religion. Any and all resentments are essentially sources of suffering and a detriment to peaceful living. If you are unclear or at odds with your feelings about God and religion, it would be best to find a way to make peace and accept that there is no one perfect path and that the ultimate goal is peace. This training manual is based on the philosophy of Omnism, and it is believed that Ego—not evil—is the cause of suffering and that if God exists, it does not judge us. Also, it is important to understand the concept of powerlessness. Powerlessness simply means that whether something is in charge of life or nothing is, we as individuals are definitely not in charge of life and without acceptance of that, we are living an illusion of control.

Being powerless, grateful, humble, and honest is the fuel required to make healthy decisions and attract better things into our lives. The next chapter teaches how to achieve those things.

7

THE SOLUTIONS

As identified by the founders of AA, the thinking that is most harmful to people is the judgment associated with character defects and resentments. Whether we are judging ourselves, other people, or any part of our experience, the act of having a judgmental mind keeps humans suspended in a constant state of bargaining and non-acceptance. Several small measures are available to willfully reprogram our thoughts into healthy, sustainable patterns. These measures were outlined by the founders of AA, and they include the twelve steps of recovery. Most of the literature of AA is in support of these new behaviors, developing improved self-care routines, and experiencing a daily reprieve as the result of surrendering to a process of recovery. It is our belief that the twelve steps were not invented; they were discovered, and that is why there are so many different ways to word them. The twelve steps are the natural way to live free from guilt, shame, regret, and remorse.

Sadly, it is often required that people suffer greatly and hit bottom before they are ready to learn and apply to a recovery program. Again, this is due to the inability of the human mind to learn new information when trapped in the bargaining stage of grieving or while closed-minded with denial. Hitting bottom, whether it is caused by an emotional crash or a massive shock to the system, means that we experience a psychic change. The reasons we need change often become clear in the tears of surrender and following emotional breakdowns. It may also occur during a near-death experience or a "Wake Up Call;" however, in each case, we change our minds from thinking we could handle something to we cannot handle the problem and need help.

It is a great blow to the human Ego to fall from grace and realize powerlessness. Whenever we experience a loss, we also experience the grieving process, and if we reach acceptance, it will mean breaking an emotional attachment to something that we once wanted. Hitting bottom represents the surrender stage of grieving and once in acceptance, we are ready to learn something new and are able to accept help from others. This represents the first step of recovery.

Attachments are often complicated and multi-dimensional. An attachment to a person, for example, is not just one thing about that person; it is a collection of things and includes the other people, places, and things associated with that person. Depending on the emotional investment and willingness to let go, grieving the loss of a person may never end or take years. Whether we are experiencing the loss ourselves or giving support to others, it is vital to acknowledge the need to be angry, cry, and isolate. The loss may feel similar to a death, but eventually, the trauma of loss is released, and life becomes manageable again. Holding back our tears keeps the trauma trapped in our systems; we need to surrender and let go before we can experience acceptance. Experiencing numerous emotional breakdowns over a single loss may be necessary, and these need to be considered a healthy, normal, and effective form of self-care.

The first three steps of recovery are meant to provide someone with a bigger and better option: a reason to change. After hitting bottom, it is important to believe that things can get better and that something besides our own thinking will give us the answers we are looking for, which is step two. Using peace as a benchmark for mental health, surrendering to peace and trusting in its healing ability represents a third step.

TO RECAP:

» I give up. I cannot do this anymore. I need help.
» There is something we can connect to that is peaceful and healthy, and it can guide us to mental health if we are willing to change.
» We make a decision to surrender to peace daily and stop fighting life.

When we are peaceful, we experience a state of awareness known as acceptance. It is very simple, very predictable, consistent, and proven. Once we are peaceful, we can look at our past, present, and future more honestly and without expectation.

The "Housecleaning Steps" are where the real work of recovery begins in what is referred to as a searching and fearless moral inventory.

For a complete online inventory process, please visit our website at www.mixedrecovery.com and look under "recovery services." There are forms that have been translated and modified from Alcoholics Anonymous, plus additional inventory work taken from a variety of sources. We encourage you to share this information with someone trusted either within our organization or with someone you know, preferably someone who understands recovery, has worked the steps themselves, and has their own sponsor. However, it is more important to feel safe with the person we share with than having someone who is an expert in recovery. In some cases, it may take several different people with whom to complete the housecleaning steps, so choose wisely and allow your intuition to guide you.

INVENTORY LISTS

Gratitude List – It is said that a grateful addict/alcoholic doesn't use. This is because the negative thoughts of our resentments and character defects are the primary cause of relapse; they create the desire to escape. It is important to recognize that when we are in active addiction of any kind, we are escaping and treating our traumas. Once free, now we will need to face the thoughts, emotions, and consequences of our past. Practicing gratitude helps to manage our emotions and the effects of PAWS (post-acute withdrawal syndrome), the tendency to obsess, and chronic negative thinking. A common recommendation is to start each day by writing out at least ten things we are grateful for and share that list with your sponsor for the first ninety days of recovery.

Resentment List – Because resentments are at the root of addiction, it is best to start processing them right away. We recommend that you begin with the most recent resentments first. Later, we can look at childhood resentments, which are deeply connected to the current-day issues we are experiencing. It is important to process each resentment, and though we may not be ready to take any action, we can begin making amends simply by becoming willing to do something someday. The resentments need to be categorized as follows:

1. What happened, and who was involved?
2. What was their part in it?
3. What was our part in it?
4. What will we do differently from now on?

Inventory of Fears – Fear is crippling and limits our ability to take action. Like with resentments, we need to inventory what the fear is, how it affects us, what our part is in the fear, and what we can do about it if anything. In some cases, there is no action that can be taken, and therefore we need to accept that what we fear may be unavoidable.

Character Weaknesses and Strengths – In many cases, our weaknesses and strengths have the same root and the difference between healthy and unhealthy is the boundaries we have set for ourselves. For example, being generous is widely considered a positive quality; however, that is no longer true if we are giving more than we can afford to. Make a list of all your qualities, healthy and unhealthy, and how you see yourself.

Sexual Conduct – A similar process is used to inventory the harm we have caused with our sexual behaviors. Please keep in mind that sponsors are not licensed professionals, and they are limited in how much of your trauma they can handle. If you have been involved in illegal sexual activities, be very careful who you share this information with and without being dishonest, limit the amount of graphic details you share. How much your sponsor or recovery partner is willing to handle is something that needs to be discussed and understood in advance. Once the boundaries are established, explain what happened, who was hurt, how they were hurt, what you will do differently from now on, and what amends you can make without causing any more harm.

Additional Harms – To become free from past regrets, we eventually need to face any harm we have caused to others. Make a list of all the people you have harmed, and allow yourself to feel how they may feel about what has happened. Become willing to make amends to all of them. The same format is applied here as with other inventory lists: who have we harmed, how did we harm them, what problems did it cause for them, and what amends can we make without causing more harm?

Seven Harmful Behaviors – The seven deadly sins are one of the models for inventory suggested by Alcoholics Anonymous. Removing the religious stigma, we call these the seven harmful behaviors and ask that you inventory what things you have done that involved the following items:

1. Pride
2. Greed
3. Lust
4. Envy
5. Gluttony
6. Wrath
7. Sloth

(More specific explanations are available on the website.)

Financial Harms – Do you have a spending addiction? Do you owe people money? Have you given away things that you could not afford to lose? Do you hoard money? Inventory all the details about your financial problems, what you have done, how it affected you, how it affected other people, and what amends you can make for these behaviors.

Childhood Traumas – This inventory practice is in addition to the standard suggestions, yet it may be the single most important. All of the problems we are experiencing in the present are deeply rooted in the past: a process called Social Conditioning. Any moments from our childhood that are marked with the emotional signature of shame are part of our traumas and create modern-day limiting beliefs until they are healed. Please create a list of every embarrassing or tragic moment that still haunts you when you think about it today. It can include any type of trauma or past regret. Were you a bully, or did someone bully you? Were you molested, beaten, or abused? Did your parents have addictions or mental health issues? Take your time, organize your thoughts, and talk about everything that still troubles you with someone safe.

Wellness and Balance – This inventory is in addition to the standard inventory items. Wellness is based on self-care, and focus is placed on relatively equal portions in eight different categories. Addicts tend to hyper-focus in a small number of areas where they receive the most pleasure and ignore other areas, sometimes completely. Describe in detail the things you do to care for yourself in the following areas:

> » *Emotional Intelligence* – Expressing and processing emotions.
> » *Physical Wellness* – Exercise, medical care, and nutrition.
> » *Socio-Cultural* – A sense of community, unity, and connectedness.
> » *Financial* – How well you make and manage your money.
> » *Environmental* – The quality and impact of the places where you spend time.
> » *Occupational* – The career you have chosen and how you occupy your time productively.
> » *Spiritual* – Honest expression of feelings and self-awareness.
> » *Intellectual* – The time you invest in learning new things.

If you find yourself crying a lot or getting upset while you work on your personal inventory, you are doing it right. The primary purpose of this work is to help us process our emotions, organize our thoughts, and complete the grieving process. After identifying and accepting both our healthy and unhealthy qualities, we are empowered to make practical changes to our behaviors, also known as "amends."

Making Amends – Once we have gotten through the mess of inventory, generally, we are more peaceful, and we feel compelled to make amends. It is not so much work as it is just letting go of what we have been doing and replacing it with a healthier, changed behavior. It is very important to understand that amends are not apologies; they are changed behaviors. Apologies are either confessions of the changed behaviors or excuses to keep acting the same way. If we feel bad about something we have done, we will naturally want to confess what we have done to the people we have harmed and let them know that we do not want to be that way anymore. However, timing and circumstance are very important factors. Making direct amends to others is only advised after we have considered how it might impact them and avoid situations where we may cause more harm.

This is the reason that willingness is more important than action. One spiritual belief, known as the law of attraction, suggests that when someone is ready to hear our confession, the situation will present itself at the correct time. How and when to make direct amends has a lot to do with what is honest for us, and we may feel strongly that we cannot live with ourselves unless we make an effort. Still, this needs to be tempered with reason. Is it too soon? Will what we say cause more harm?

In the cases where making direct amends is ill-advised or no longer possible, there is a practice we suggest to help you gain closure. Write a letter that you do not send. Write a letter to each of the people you wish you could talk to but cannot for one of many possible reasons: because it is a bad idea, you cannot find them, they do not want to hear from you, they are deceased, etc. Say everything that you wish you could in person, in your writing. Tell them everything that you feel, what you did, how it affected you, and what you have learned, and ask for forgiveness. Ultimately, we are writing the letter to ourselves, yet there is something profound when we express ourselves in writing; it heals us. You may want to edit the letter a number of times until it says exactly what you feel, and then you have the option of either sharing it with your sponsor or destroying the letter as an expression of letting go.

In the *AA Big Book* p83-84, there are specific promises regarding how our lives improve when we go through the housecleaning steps. At the end of that passage, a bold statement is made about these promises, "They will always materialize if we work for them."

It has been discovered that the only times recovery does not provide results is when people are unwilling or unable to surrender to the program.

Having completed the painful journey of cleaning out negativity, we need a process to replace past behaviors and keep us on track and honest. In the maintenance steps (steps ten through twelve), people tune into how to continue their growth and remain balanced. The subconscious mind is powerful, and without maintenance, we risk falling back into old behaviors.

8
DAILY REPRIEVE

Once the house cleaning steps have been completed, the bargaining mind has become mostly quiet or at least manageable, and now we transition to maintenance. The subconscious mind contains billions of emotional subroutines that can lure us back into old harmful behaviors; therefore, maintaining daily self-awareness and recovery practices will prevent those behaviors from becoming dominant again. The daily reprieve consists of a number of things that may not come naturally for people, and that will need commitment and consistency. It is up to each of us to find the wisdom to commit to our personal growth and self-awareness.

Spiritual maintenance includes a combination of these options:

- » Prayer, journaling, or talking to ourselves.
- » Meditation.
- » Gratitude.
- » Selflessness and service work.
- » Fearless honesty and promptly admitting our wrongs.
- » Crying as needed.
- » Being part of a support community.
- » Periods of isolation and continued daily self-reflection and inventory.

Prayer – For people who have issues with God or religion, please consider the act of prayer as the process of talking to yourself in your most honest and sincere manner. Is there a god listening? That cannot be proven, so "God" cannot be the healing factor. The healing element is the honest confession, which we do by talking to ourselves, journaling, or praying. We need to be honest with ourselves before we can be honest with other people. It has also been suggested that if the idea of God is an issue, make an imaginary friend to talk to.

It is against the principles of our organization to try and convince, convert, or corrupt anyone's concept of a higher power. We do, however, suggest that a non-judgmental environment is the healthiest and easiest to be completely honest in. We also recommend the following prayer practices for those who are willing:

» Admitting our faults and asking to have them removed.
» Asking for guidance and expressing a willingness to change.
» Expressing gratitude.
» Confession.

More than anything, daily prayer is capable of preparing us for the day and can reduce our tendency to overthink. Remember that the real sickness of addiction is overthinking; relying on a higher power can drastically reduce our desire to ruminate or worry.

Meditation – This is widely misunderstood. Sleeping is a form of meditation. So is listening to music, watching TV, practicing tai chi, participating in endurance sports, playing video games, or fishing under the right conditions. Meditation occurs any time we remove ourselves from logic, will, and desire. If we can quiet or replace our thoughts, we leave the bargaining stage of grieving and become more present. This is important because, more often than not, it is the peaceful part of our existence that holds the answers that we seek. In the silence of deep meditation, Ego cannot exist, and from that perspective, it is easier to let go of our attachments and gain perspective.

Gratitude – Practicing gratitude generates healthy opportunities for change. Being and expressing gratitude tunes the human mind into healthier thinking, habits, and personal connections. Misery loves company, so negative minds gravitate toward each other; meanwhile, grateful minds attract opportunities. Becoming grateful may be a difficult task while we are in the depths of anger, depression, and obsession. Yet, practicing gratitude is one of the first things suggested to newcomers because it is widely known that grateful addicts/alcoholics do not continue to use.

Making a gratitude list is a common suggestion, listing at least ten things daily, and it is recommended that we keep this practice going for up to ninety days and no less than twenty-one days.

Selflessness and Service Work – Humans are at their best when they are selfless in service to others. Without service work, there is a dimension of life that is completely missed, which is also a basic human need in the area of wellness called self-awareness. There are many forms and opportunities for service work, including sponsoring other people in recovery. The twelfth step of recovery describes a need that we never realized we had. Working all the steps of recovery causes many people to experience a spiritual awakening where they no longer question the steps; they have changed their lives to include them. They also become compelled to give support to those who are still struggling and share what they have learned during the recovery process. That is one of the impressive things about the twelve steps; if completed with sincerity, they become self-propagating.

Prior to completing the steps, people in recovery may have a desire to help in ways other than sponsorship. Before completion, we can still become accountability partners for others by being safe to talk to. Other service work includes activities that are common with attending meetings like making coffee, passing out literature, cleaning and organizing, and performing some of the readings that are common at the beginning of meetings. Service work does not need to be limited to recovery; it can include religious organizations, charities, and social groups.

Fearless honesty and promptly admitting our wrongs – Humans are flawed, and one of our biggest mistakes is expecting ourselves to be perfect. Promptly admitting our faults protects us from the sickness of living a lie. Anything that we need to hide is a source of unhealthy thoughts, and so returning to peace means unloading any guilt, shame, or remorse as it happens. The consequences of telling the truth are almost always less than the consequences of lies. While in an active addiction, lying, cheating, stealing, sneaking, and hiding are very common behaviors. Recovery is honesty training, and once we are in the habit of being completely honest, it is difficult to live with ourselves when we are not.

Crying as needed – Crying is how humans release trauma and is one of the most direct methods for increasing our levels of acceptance. Life is suffering, and when we are not suffering, other people still are and so life hurts from time to time. We are conditioned to "suck it up," "walk it off," "grow up," "man up," "pull up our big girl pants," and other repressive expressions. Sadly, trauma does not leave our systems, and without crying when we need to, we only increase our levels of denial. Learn to allow yourself to cry and realize that tears are temporary, but the effects of denial are long-term and damaging.

Being part of a support community – Whether it is a religious group, a book club, a recovery fellowship, or a community effort, being among like-minded people is an important part of living a balanced life. In the company of people who understand and support us, we remember who we are, find opportunities for service, and remain grounded. Recovery fellowships can be especially beneficial when there are people who are serious about their recovery and practice using the concept of acceptance.

Periods of isolation and continued daily self-reflection and inventory – Humans need time and space to process grief and organize our thoughts. It is in these times that we learn the most about ourselves. It is especially important to find time to be alone when we are in committed relationships and when we are raising children. Having private time in the morning and evening is a healthy way to reflect on the day ahead of or behind us and determine if we need to adjust any behaviors or make amends. Without this time, it is easy to enter into an automatic mode where we risk returning to old patterns.

Developing a daily reprieve is more effective when combined with complete wellness. Often, we are focused on a few areas of our lives intently and neglect other areas of our lives. Developing an understanding of what completes our wellness gives us additional tools for positive change.

9

FORMULAS AND PATTERNS

To ease the process of reprogramming our minds, small formulas, patterns, and universal truths can form lasting corrective attachments. Alcoholics Anonymous famously promotes "One day at a time." This statement is also taught by Jesus and Buddha in their own language, and it is a reminder to have faith in life and avoid obsessing; just focus on what is in front of us. Similarly, in my own language, I would like to share things that I have found to be universally true. I use these phrases whenever I am experiencing negativity in my life as a reminder to remain peaceful, honest, and accountable.

- » Every accusation is a confession.
- » Expectations are resentments waiting to happen.
- » If I am bargaining (obsessing/complaining), I need to let go of something.
- » If it causes harm, let go.
- » When we let go of what is harmful, something better replaces it.
- » Anything that follows the word "I" is the Ego describing the Ego.
- » We are peace.
- » Anything that is not peaceful is Ego.
- » Ego is logic, will, and desire – our collection of attachments.

» All defensive emotional responses are an indication of denial.
» We are never right; we are either attached or learning.
» Suffering ends when we accept it.
» Surrender/crying is a proven cure for anger, bargaining, anxiety, and depression.
» Denial is a lack of emotional intelligence.
» Humans are always grieving, whether we are aware of it or not.
» Comfort is an Ego trap; coping is the process of authentic life.
» Bragging is like begging for losses.
» Gratitude is the energy of creation.
» The subconscious mind is more powerful than willpower.
» Let go of outcomes, detach from plans, show up, and be present.
» Life is incomplete without being of service to others.
» At our core, we all have the same moral code.
» We attract people, places, and situations of matching dysfunction until we heal the parts of us that need them.

10
PROS AND CONS OF
RECOVERY

There is something that occurs within a number of people who remain in recovery: a psychic change where they realize a number of important truths. We come to know that acceptance really is the cure for most of life's challenges: if not immediate, then eventual. We understand the need to give and receive acceptance and the importance of sharing what we have learned with others who are suffering as we have.

There are many ways to carry the message, and anyone who has worked the steps with a sponsor can be a sponsor themselves. The gift we receive from giving support is one of the basic principles of recovery, and often, the sponsor gets more benefit from the relationship than the sponsee. This training manual attempts to put the steps of recovery into a language that makes sense for most people with the goal of creating not only more qualified sponsors for people in recovery but also high-functioning members of the general public.

One of the limiting factors of recovery is that sponsorship is nonprofessional and, most often, free. Because it is free, it is not taken very seriously. Also, there are a limited number of qualified sponsors because the process is time-consuming and unpaid efforts can eventually become a burden. Finally, until now there has been no organization willing or able to train people to be sponsors. This is why we intend to take sponsorship to another level by providing training that allows people to have both paying clients and give free sponsorship to people in recovery. There is a very simple guideline we intend to follow: we will advertise and market for clients from the general public but give free sponsorship to the people we meet in a recovery fellowship. This way we are not crossing any lines or violating any traditions. The reality is that most of the people who are introduced to twelve-step recovery are frightened off by any number of factors and so there is a much larger market outside of twelve-step meetings than inside. For example, it is estimated that only two to eight percent of the people introduced to AA will get a sponsor and complete the steps. Most will drop out of recovery, claiming it did not work for them.

Twelve-step recovery does not work for everyone for one simple reason: not everyone is willing to work the steps. Also, there are a number of Ego traps in recovery that can trigger people and give a false impression of what it means to be in recovery. To help you navigate recovery and understand why you may feel safer with some people than others, this training manual includes a list of common behaviors found at recovery meetings. *As always, every accusation is a confession so admittedly, I have been all of these things in varying degrees myself. Each of the following items is a common Ego trap, both in recovery, religion, and life.*

Pink Cloud – When recovery starts to make sense, and people experience the immediate benefits of acceptance, they enter a phase of recovery where they become blissful and full of hope. This stage is often short-lived and may lead to the next relapse. The pink cloud is often but not always a short-lived stage of increased faith, followed by new addictions and obsessions or a return to old addictions, with an increase of denial. Please note: when newcomers suddenly find God, they may become obsessive, compulsive, and unbalanced. When the state of euphoria passes, and they realize life is still difficult at times, they may become discouraged and relapse. It is very important to encourage people to remain grounded and remind them that the pink cloud is just one of the things we experience in recovery.

Dry Drunk – Recovery is littered with people who have hit bottom and broken their obsession with alcohol, drugs or other addictions but are otherwise just going through the motions. They have not learned how to completely surrender their Ego to recovery. One of the most destructive thoughts in recovery is, "I got this." The reality is we never get it, never had it, and do not want it because what we are describing is the illusion of control. Dry drunks may become Big Book Thumpers and really frighten off anyone who is not willing to memorize the literature provided in recovery. Dry drunk is a term that applies globally to anyone who has broken the obsession for a primary addiction, yet continue to hold on to character defects and resentments.

Big Book Thumpers – Every religion and major recovery fellowship has its own approved literature, and the books are often brilliant, and many people study them. This in itself is a positive force, and for people who enjoy reading, we recommend this practice for whatever fellowship you are involved in. Not everyone is interested in this process, and it is not a requirement for recovery. The problem arises when the people who are well-versed in the literature get the idea that they are doing it the right way, the only way, or better than the people who are not. Often, these people have unresolved control issues, and they can be a very negative force in recovery as well, having a big book answer for everything and using their knowledge as a weapon to put other people in their place.

Control Freak – The control freak has an awful case of the "shoulds." They have found a lifestyle that is manageable for them, and now they feel it is the right way to do it. When they share, it often sounds like a massive list of things that we must do in order for our recovery to be valid. This is, of course, untrue; recovery looks different for everyone. What is really happening is they are expressing all the things that they need to do for themselves, and it has become another addiction for them.

Guru Complex – People who believe that there is only one possible way and that they are doing it often correct others and have a number of reasons why this behavior is justified.

Better-Than Complex – Some people believe it is possible to be better than other people and experience judgmental thought patterns. Often, when an opportunity is presented, they gain satisfaction from pointing out other people's flaws and then taking "the high road" to show how they are better than the person who they have insulted. In reality, all people are equal and there is no way to measure the goodness or badness in humans.

Spiritual Complex – There are some misconceptions about what it means to be spiritual. Some people say that religion is for people who fear hell, and spirituality is for people who have been there. Some people may proudly boast that they are "spiritual, not religious." It is the position of our organization that there are distinct benefits to many religious practices and that spirituality may absolutely be attained by people of any faith or none. Being against religion is short-sighted, and being vocal about it is practicing nonacceptance and bigotry. Religion itself is not the issue. As stated earlier, the real issue is Ego. There are both unhealthy and healthy teachings in any belief system or religion, and we support people who seek and practice the peaceful, humble, and accepting aspects of their faith.

Logic Complex – Ego is logic, will, and desire. This means everything we think, do, and want is part of our Ego. Logic complex is a condition that happens to many people who consider science, facts, and reason to be a type of higher power. When logic is a higher power, there is not much room for the spiritual dimension of life. Still, this manual attempts to explain spiritual concepts in a logical manner that may appeal to a broader audience, provided they have an open mind.

Holistic Complex – The word spirituality has many meanings for many different people. We prefer to replace that word with the clearer and more descriptive expression "honest and self-aware." Many people believe that spiritual practices lead to enlightenment, and we wholeheartedly disagree. Self-awareness is a process of identifying and letting go of the harmful beliefs and behaviors we have as individuals. Yoga, meditation, crystals, and horoscopes may hold some keys to this process; however, they are not even close to replacing the revelations we experience when working on a formal recovery program with a sponsor.

Comfort Trap – Many times in recovery, when it stops hurting, we become comfortable and stop seeking answers. For example, many people stay clean and sober by simply attending meetings and/or reading literature. If clean and sober is the only concern, this approach is fine. Recovery, however, is about personal growth and accountability, so even after we complete the steps, it does not mean that we are done with them. This is one of the main reasons why part of our spiritual maintenance includes a continued personal inventory.

Spiritual / Religious Addiction – In any group or community, aside from the newcomers, the fanatics are generally the sickest members. The Guru Complex, Better-Than Complex, Big Book

Thumpers and other Ego traps may be signs of religious or spiritual addictions. Humans are creatures of habit, and for many people, changing addictions may be the best they can do. Sadly, differences in beliefs often cause major problems in society and are factors in many wars. Please remember that acceptance of everyone and everything is a primary principle of recovery. It is our belief that true enlightenment is the utter absence of attachments, so replacing one set of attachments for another really does not qualify as a benchmark for mental health.

11

INTO ACTION / TIPS FOR SPONSORS

The process for recovery and the process for training to become a sponsor are one and the same. However, this training manual expands on a number of topics and is designed to give you specific advantages over the average person in recovery. It also teaches a number of concepts that are not found in any other recovery program, yet they will aid you in your progress in any fellowship. They will also provide you with enough knowledge and original information that you will be empowered to charge the general public for paid sponsorship. As mentioned previously, this course supports the idea of having both paid clients and continuing to provide service work for people who are struggling.

The reasons for both are simple. Many people who enter into recovery are on a losing streak. They may be losing their homes, jobs, families, and possessions as a result of their addictions. Trying to charge people who are hitting bottom is unethical and impractical. At the same time, there are many people who are high functioning and have no interest in attending twelve-step meetings but still need the kind of emotional support that only a sponsor can provide.

As sponsors, we are more likely to respond to a crisis call immediately, have flexible schedules, and be willing to give people emotional support in their most desperate hours without an appointment. This level of commitment deserves compensation and accepting donations for our efforts is entirely reasonable and plausible because of our training and the value of service. With those things in mind, this chapter is likely one of the most important in the book because it covers precisely how to be an effective sponsor from start to finish.

STEP ONE: FINDING OUT IF THEY HAVE HIT BOTTOM

Real recovery does not begin until people have accepted that they have a problem and that they need help. The language people use and their behaviors are normally pretty clear indicators if they are ready to begin, yet be aware that often, once people start to feel better, they assume they are doing better, and that is when they are likely to relapse. Watch for the signs of the surrender stage of grieving because this is when people are normally desperate enough to try anything. They may also have reached the acceptance stage and are experiencing some clean time, at which point they may become willing to continue the process. Listen for expressions like, "I can't," "I need help," "I do not want to do this anymore," "If I do not stop, I am going to lose everything," and "I am ready and would appreciate your help."

As a standard practice, if it sounds like they are hitting bottom, ask if they are able to cry and if they have been crying lately. Not all spiritual awakenings happen with tears; some are more like rude awakenings that snap us into awareness. However, if people have been crying a lot, that is a good sign. Encourage them to keep doing that as much as they need to, and explain that it is how we release trauma.

STEP TWO: ESTABLISH A BASIS OF FAITH

Ask the potential sponsee about their basis of faith and if they have a higher power. No matter how they respond, learn to respect and stick to that belief system. It is against company policy to convert people. However, if and only if they ask for help deciding, you may explain your own belief system and see if that would work for them. Generally speaking, we are most effective with people when we can match their language and religious interests.

STEP THREE: CHECK WILLINGNESS

Many people want to recover or break an addiction. Unfortunately, not many of them are willing to do what is necessary. At twelve-step meetings, we hear "meeting makers make it," and to some degree, that is true. The reason for this is because at tables we can find the fellowship and acceptance we need to live more balanced lives. Unfortunately, remaining clean or sober is only the first step in recovery, and without taking the rest of the steps seriously, people generally fall into Ego traps and level off, or even worse, relapse.

As a sponsor, it is imperative for our own well-being to know when someone is serious about their recovery and will not waste our time or damage our peace trying to help them. The biggest signs of a sponsee who is not ready are these behaviors:

They will:

» Want to argue or split hairs with the information that is being presented.
» Say one thing and do something different.
» Challenge or ignore our boundaries.
» Ask for money, cigarettes, and inappropriate favors.
» Start talking like they "got it" and know what they are doing.
» Offer unsolicited advice.

» Judge us, take our inventory, or question our recovery.
» Use non-recovery-related information to challenge recovery.
» Make excuses for their behaviors.
» Blame everyone and everything but themselves.
» Give you lip service; tell you what you want to hear instead of what you need to hear.
» Relapse instead of calling.
» Play the victim.
» Claim they have already tried everything and nothing works.
» Display a lack of commitment and consistency.
» Come up with other solutions that have nothing to do with recovery.
» Avoid the fourth step inventory work completely.

To help determine who is capable of committing themselves to recovery, ask your sponsee what things they are willing to do for their recovery.

The most common things include:

» Attending twelve-step meetings, online or in person.
» Working the twelve steps.
» Working with a sponsor.
» Becoming a sponsor once they complete the steps.
» Read recovery literature.
» Prayer and or meditation.
» Journaling.
» Complete the fourth step inventory.
» Improve self-care.
» Practice powerlessness.
» Practice fearless honesty and radical acceptance.
» Perform service work either at meetings or for the general public.
» Read scripture or self-help books.

» Cry: experience the painful feelings of letting go.
» Talk to someone safe about past traumas and options for healing.
» Practice daily routines for spiritual maintenance and self-awareness.

Please remember that saying is not doing. If someone is willing and takes some of our recovery suggestions, consider it a blessing because many people do not. Change is very difficult for many people, and so it is important to remove all expectations. At the same time, be aware of when a sponsee or client is simply not ready and, basically, need to hurt themselves some more before they become ready.

You may or may not be the type of sponsor who feels strongly about reading recovery literature. Be aware, not everyone is willing to do a lot of reading and so there are potential mismatches in sponsorship because of the difference in reading willingness. This can be said of each of the options available in recovery; many people do not want to go to meetings, and many people are not willing to pray. These things alone do not mean that they cannot be helped. The important thing is that they are willing to do at least some of the practices of recovery. If they are not, then they may not be ready, or recovery is just not an option for them. Be willing to let go of a sponsee or client if they do not have any willingness. Explain to them why and let them know if they ever become ready, you will be there. Recovery has an open-door policy, and they are welcome back even though they may need to try a different sponsor, one they will listen to.

STEP FOUR: FEARLESS INVENTORY

Many people will exercise steps one through three and never go beyond. That is absolutely fine; let them do that. The people who are willing to move forward are the ones who benefit most from a sponsor. For your convenience, an entire inventory process has been posted on our website at https://mixedrecovery.com/recovery-services.

This process will be added to and improved over time to help reach more people and give support for more conditions and programs. You are not required to stick to this format, and please be advised that every fellowship has its own inventory process. The Mixed Recovery, Inc. inventory process is loosely based on the suggestions for Alcoholics Anonymous, with certain enhancements intended to give a more complete picture of wellness and balance. The questions asked are meant to be thought-provoking and may be much different than people are accustomed to; each of them is self-awareness related. Fearless honesty is key when completing an inventory process; however, we recommend that the process is done more than once in a lifetime and with each pass, we take a deeper look at who we are.

STEP FIVE: CONFESSION

This is where the real value of a sponsor becomes clear. We are meant to be the safest person a sponsee has to talk to. We never judge; we validate and relate. We do not give advice or directions; we share suggestions for the things that we have worked for us. We listen more than we talk, and when appropriate, we share confessions of our own to keep the relationship equal. Sponsees may share things that we have never experienced and cannot relate to, yet we can still empathize with them. We recommend that as sponsors for Mixed Recovery, Inc., we take the time to read everything that a sponsee or client has been willing to journal or submit in a form.

STEPS SIX AND SEVEN: WILLINGNESS AND LETTING GO

These are ongoing themes throughout recovery. It is important to note that we can become willing to let something go, even when we really do not want to. Resentments, in particular, can be tricky and take a long time to heal. Character weaknesses may be deeply embedded and will require a lot of patience to heal as well. For example, we may decide to quit smoking, be convinced that we need to, and talk about how we are going to, but addictions can be very difficult to break. Until such a time comes that we actually let go of a behavior, we can work on willingness and be kind to ourselves in the process. Making changes in our behaviors comes down to a single factor: harm. If the behavior is causing us or someone else harm, we need to modify it or let it go completely.

Prayer is one effective means to become willing, and if that is one of the activities your sponsee or client will commit to, ask them to pray daily, asking to have the resentment or character weakness taken from them until it happens. Another means of becoming willing is journaling all the harm that we are causing and experiencing with the negative behaviors.

STEP EIGHT: AMENDS LIST

The amends list is intended to be a reference source and a manner to organize our thoughts and prepare us for changing other behaviors. In the case of drinking, staying sober is automatically one amend. Apologies may not be necessary. It depends entirely on the situation. In truth, an apology is either a confession of something we do not want to do anymore or an excuse to keep doing it. In many cases, people do not want to hear another apology from us, and it will not help anyway. The interesting thing about step eight is that it is more important to become willing to make an amend than it is to take action. When we match the energy, the universe will align things for us, and the opportunity will just happen.

STEP NINE: DIRECT AMENDS

As mentioned previously, direct amends may not be needed or possible, and suggestions have already been offered on how to handle that potentiality. In the event that direct amends are needed, and it makes sense to proceed, this is a formula that is effective:

» Admit and confess to what we have done and do not want to do anymore.
» Ask how it affected the other person, and have them tell us what we did wrong.
» Ask what we can do to make up for it.
» Do it.

All of this is assuming you are ready and want to continue having a relationship with the other person. When making direct amends, prepare yourself for any possible outcome. With the very best of intentions and the most carefully selected words, we may still get a negative response and even make the situation worse. It happens. Detach and accept in advance that we cannot control the outcome, and anything is possible. How other people respond to our efforts is not as important as making the effort. Prepare your sponsees or clients with these simple facts and be ready to support them no matter what happens.

STEPS TEN THROUGH TWELVE: THE MAINTENANCE STEPS

One simple truth about recovery is that we are never cured of anything. We are given a daily reprieve based on the maintenance of our spiritual condition. This means that, provided we continue to take recovery seriously and incorporate some form of recovery in our daily activities, we can place our conditions in remission. If we stop actively recovering, then there is a definite risk of returning to old behaviors, especially in the event of some new trauma or tragedy in our lives. The end game for us and the people we work with is to create and maintain new healthy behaviors that will keep us safe from relapse. Teaching our sponsees and clients to take a daily inventory is much easier when we practice it ourselves. Also, the benefits of prayer or meditation are easily explained by people who practice them daily. Finally, engaging in service work and being a part of some type of community is very beneficial and an effective way to maintain our spiritual fitness.

Mixed Recovery, Inc. specifically markets to people who are not likely to attend twelve-step meetings. In fact, it is against company policy to solicit clients from twelve-step groups. At the same time, we want our trained sponsors to attend meetings and sponsor people for free if they are willing. For the people we attract who are not in recovery, it is okay to recommend or suggest different fellowships, and there is no conflict of interest, provided that is not where we met them.

Please keep in mind that although we maintain nonprofessional status, this does not mean it cannot become a career or that we do not know what we are doing. In terms of company policy, it means for the safety of our trained sponsors, they are allowed to let go of any client or sponsee they want with no risk of penalties from the company. We ask that you try to remain polite, though we understand if you do not. Mixed Recovery, Inc. understands that we deal with people who have different levels of self-awareness, and many of the people we work with may have toxic or abusive behaviors. Because the company screens for narcissism and is seeking people who are specifically empaths, we also understand there is a need to protect our staff from emotional abuse and support our members in their right to decline service to anyone at any time without explanation. We leave coddling and the restrictions of appropriate behavior to the professionals.

12

MANIFESTING

As mentioned previously, Mixed Recovery, Inc. recognizes and is based on things that are considered universal truths and rejects any science that does not support these concepts. We are convinced that the universe is far stranger than we are taught in school and that the law of attraction is far more responsible for the circumstances and happenings in our lives than education and hard work will ever be. We are not suggesting that education and hard work have no value. It is our belief that those things alone are no way to live because we may be learning and doing things that really do not matter in terms of personal success, balance, wellness, and finding our true purpose in life.

Supporting the concept of the law of attraction, we present this brief description of how to manifest people, places, things, and situations into our lives. We recognize and offer the following steps as universal truth and a means to improve our lives.

BASHAR'S SEVEN STEPS OF MANIFESTING

- » *Vision* – Visualize what you want.
- » *Desire* – Be intensely excited about what you're visualizing.
- » *Belief* – Believe what you desire is possible to manifest.

> » *Acceptance* – Accept your belief and your ability to manifest it as being true.
> » *Intend* – Wanting is not enough; we must have the intention to manifest our desires.
> » *Action* – Act and behave as though your desire has already manifested; become the new you.
> » *Allowance* – Detach from any specific outcomes. The things we desire and what we receive often look very different. What we receive will be beyond expectation so hold no expectations, only feelings of gratitude.

The law of attraction is very real and always working. The reason humans have difficulty manifesting is trauma-related. First, what we want needs to be believable for us, and we need to believe we deserve it. Knowing it and doing it are very different things. After working the steps of recovery, trauma and shame have been diminished, and our abilities to manifest have increased. Learning acceptance and its partner detachment, people will begin to recognize more synchronicity in their lives and the things we need begin to appear often without explanation. This is one of the gifts and promises of the twelve steps, "we will intuitively know how to handle situations which used to baffle us." The reason for this is that working the steps leaves us with fewer things to think about.

If and when we have trouble manifesting things, then it is important to recognize that the root causes may be limiting beliefs and traumas we have not yet fully healed. Stay close to your recovery and be constantly willing to admit there is room for improvement and eventually, manifesting will become your second nature.

ABOUT THE AUTHOR

My name is Jeff, and I am not a professional. I am an alcoholic, addict, codependent, and reformed criminal with PTSD and bipolar disorder in recovery. In my life, I have either had myself or been exposed to most forms of mental illness. I have personally experienced anxiety, depression, rage, mania, schizophrenia, and Stockholm syndrome. Currently, all of those conditions are in remission because I am committed to working a daily recovery program. I do not think about the process much anymore; I just find myself doing it as needed.

No doctors, no pills, and no therapists have ever come close to the benefits I have experienced working the steps and participating in various fellowships.

In 2017, in my fifties, I experienced a psychotic break when, over the course of ten nights, I recalled a childhood that had been blocked out by hypnotherapy in my teens. Suddenly, being forced to deal with childhood traumas that I had not thought about for my entire adult life was too much for me, and I became very sick. Filled with rage and trauma, I began attacking people, friends, family, coworkers, and past clients. I have a therapist who has a restraining order against me, and I was given a police escort after I threatened a Friend of the Court judge.

I lost almost everything as a result of my traumas and the impact they had on my mind. Over the course of six years, I found myself moving around, sometimes packing up in the middle of the night and going to a new location because of a bipolar episode that destroyed the living and working relationships I had at the time.

I have been to nine different therapists in my life and known several others, and none of them had the information I needed or was looking for. Thankfully, I was in recovery at the time I became sick and stayed in recovery this entire time. Online, I eventually met Selyna Breeze, a trauma specialist in Belgium whose Rapid Transformation Therapy treatments helped me break my obsession with anger. Now, I am grateful to say that I have learned so much about myself and recovery that I cannot imagine ever wasting my time with mental health professionals again. They are still looking for answers; in recovery, we have already found them, and it is just a matter of committing and surrendering ourselves to the process.

If you or someone you love is struggling with anger, depression, anxiety, addiction, or traumas of any kind, please consider joining us in the process of recovery. It is not a matter of whether or not it works; even under the worst of circumstances, recovery can improve our lives. The real question is, have you hurt enough yet? If you are sick and tired of being sick and tired, if you want relief and are willing to go to any lengths to get it, please join the millions of people who swear by this process, and we will give you all the support we can on your journey to better, healthier days. Thank you.

Sincerely,
Rev. Jeff Rounds
Omnist Reverend and Sponsor for Mixed Recovery, Inc.

www.ingramcontent.com/pod-product-compliance
Lightning Source LLC
Chambersburg PA
CBHW072210090426
42740CB00012B/2465